Cervical Cancer

All you need to know

Dr. Sheila Harrison

Disclaimer

This content serves to provide general information about the disease and aims to empower you to seek prompt medical assistance if necessary to prevent complications. It's essential to stress that this information is not a substitute for consulting a qualified physician. The field of medical science is continually evolving, and due to the dynamic nature of medical knowledge, we recommend seeking expert advice if you encounter any inconsistencies or intend to take action based on the information in this content. Never disregard professional medical guidance or delay treatment based on something you've read online, including this material, or from any other online source. Always remember that the internet cannot cure you; rather, healing comes through the guidance of medical professionals and the providence of God.

NOTICE: *Reader Discretion is Advised due to nature of some of the image Content Of the book. Thank You.*

Table of Contents

Disclaimer 1

Table of Contents 2

Introduction 3

Section 1 4

   The Cervix 4

Section 2 5

   Types of Cervical Cancer 5

Section 3 6

   Symptoms of cervical cancer 6

Section 4 9

   Causes and Risk Factors 9

Section 5 11

   Cervical Cancer Diagnosis 11

Section 6 14

   Cervical Cancer Treatment - Briefing 14

   Detailed Clinical Approaches to Cervical Cancer
Treatment & Management 15

Section 7 33

   Prevention of Cervical Cancer 33

Section 8 36

   Myths and Facts about Cervical Cancer 36

      First Steps to Taking Care of Your Cervical
Health 47

Section 9 49

   FAQs on Cervical Cancer 49

Introduction

Cervical cancer is the third most common malignancy in women worldwide. The incidence of invasive cervical cancer has declined steadily in the United States over the past few decades; however, it remains at high levels in many developing countries. The change in the epidemiologic trend in the United States has been attributed to mass screening with Papanicolaou (Pap) tests, which permits detection and treatment of preinvasive disease.

Recognition of the etiologic role of human papillomavirus (HPV) infection in cervical cancer has led to the recommendation of adding HPV testing to the screening regimen in women 30-65 years of age (see Workup). However, women who have symptoms, abnormal screening test results, or a gross lesion of the cervix are best evaluated with colposcopy and biopsy.

Section 1

The Cervix

The cervix is the lower part or neck of the uterus [the organ in a woman's abdomen where a baby develops when she is pregnant], which connects the uterus to the vagina [the passage leading from the cervix to the outside of the body]. The cancer development in the cells lining the cervix [the lining of the lower part of the uterus that opens into the vagina] refers to cervical cancer, which is one of the most common types of cancer among females worldwide.

The development of cervical cancer may happen due to Human Papilloma Virus (HPV) infection [a virus that is spread through sexual contact or even through normal contact and can cause changes in the cells of the cervix]. It transmits through sexual contact and causes mutations in cervical cells when infected.

Though very common in the reproductive age group in females, cancer development can be easily prevented if vaccination and early screening of the disease are done. In this article, we will discuss symptoms, causes, risk factors, and other aspects of cervical cancer.

Section 2

Types of Cervical Cancer

Cervical cancer can be classified into three types based on the type of cervical cells affected:

- **Squamous cell carcinoma:** This type of cancer develops in the flat-lining cells of the cervix.
- **Adenocarcinoma:** This form of cancer originates in the mucus-secreting cells of the cervix.
- **Mixed carcinoma:** In some cases, both types of cells may be involved in cancer development.

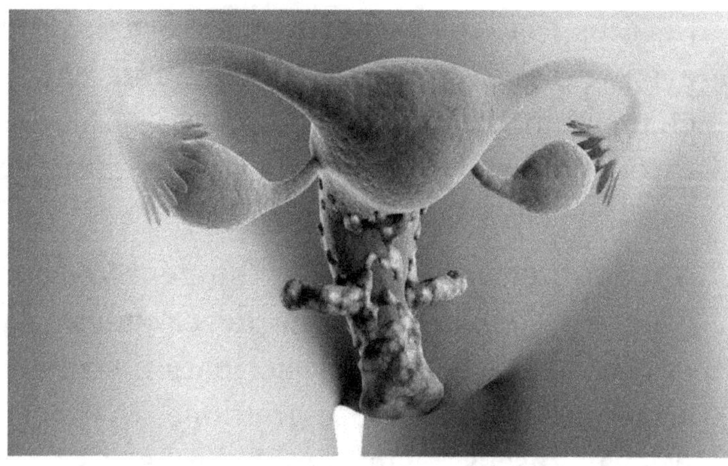

Section 3

Symptoms of cervical cancer

Cervical cancer originates in the cervix, the lowest part of the uterus that connects to the vagina. This type of cancer is primarily triggered by specific strains of the human papillomavirus (HPV), which is a sexually transmitted infection. HPV can infiltrate the protective environment of the vagina, leading to an infection.Since cervical cancer is connected to a sexually transmitted infection, it's essential to prioritize good feminine hygiene. But what does that involve? Vaginal hygiene largely depends on your age. The key is to maintain a healthy vaginal environment by preserving the right acidity levels and ensuring that your vaginal discharge remains consistent without any unusual odors.

The vagina naturally has an acidic environment, typically with a pH range of 3.8 to 4.5. This acidity helps prevent bacterial and fungal infections. Additionally, the vagina regularly discharges dead cervical and vaginal cells from the body. However, if you notice an unusual discharge or experience a change in vaginal odor,

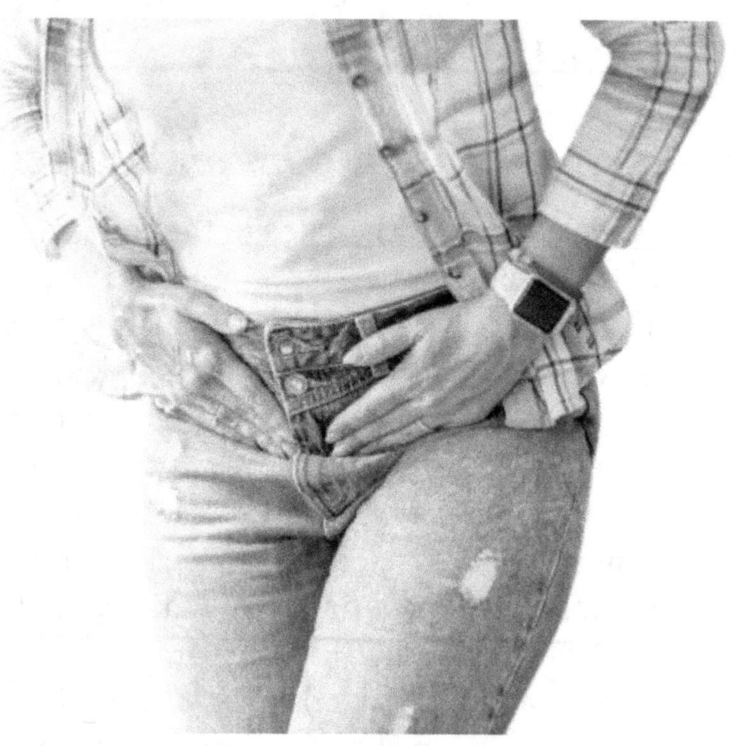

It's important to consult a doctor. Sometimes, signs of cervical cancer can appear when a healthy vaginal routine isn't maintained.

- Bleeding after sex, a pelvic exam, or douching.

- An unhealthy diet.

- Bleeding after your period.

- Very heavy periods.

- More vaginal discharge or a different odor.

- Bleeding after menopause (when your periods have stopped).
- Pain in your pelvic or lower back.
- Pain during sex.
- White discharge.
- A lot of foul-smelling vaginal discharge.
- Pain in your lower abdomen.

If you experience these symptoms and are unsure about your feminine hygiene, it's best to consult a gynecologist. Cervical cancer can be treated if caught early. Don't hesitate to describe your symptoms to the doctor, even if they don't seem severe.

Section 4

Causes and Risk Factors

Cervical cancer is primarily caused by an infection of the Human Papilloma Virus (HPV), which leads to mutations in cervical cells, potentially resulting in cancer. It's important to note that not everyone infected with HPV will develop cancer. In about 95% of cases, HPV may cause genital warts, which usually resolve on their own. However, in the remaining 5% of cases, it can lead to cell changes and the development of cancer.

Several factors increase the risk of HPV infection:

- Engaging in sexual activity with multiple partners.
- Early sexual exposure before the age of 16.
- Using birth control pills for an extended period, typically more than 5 years.
- Having a weakened immune system.
- A history of smoking.
- Multiple pregnancies or early pregnancies.

- Not using condoms during sexual intercourse.

- A family history of cervical cancer.

These factors can elevate the risk of HPV infection and, consequently, cervical cancer.

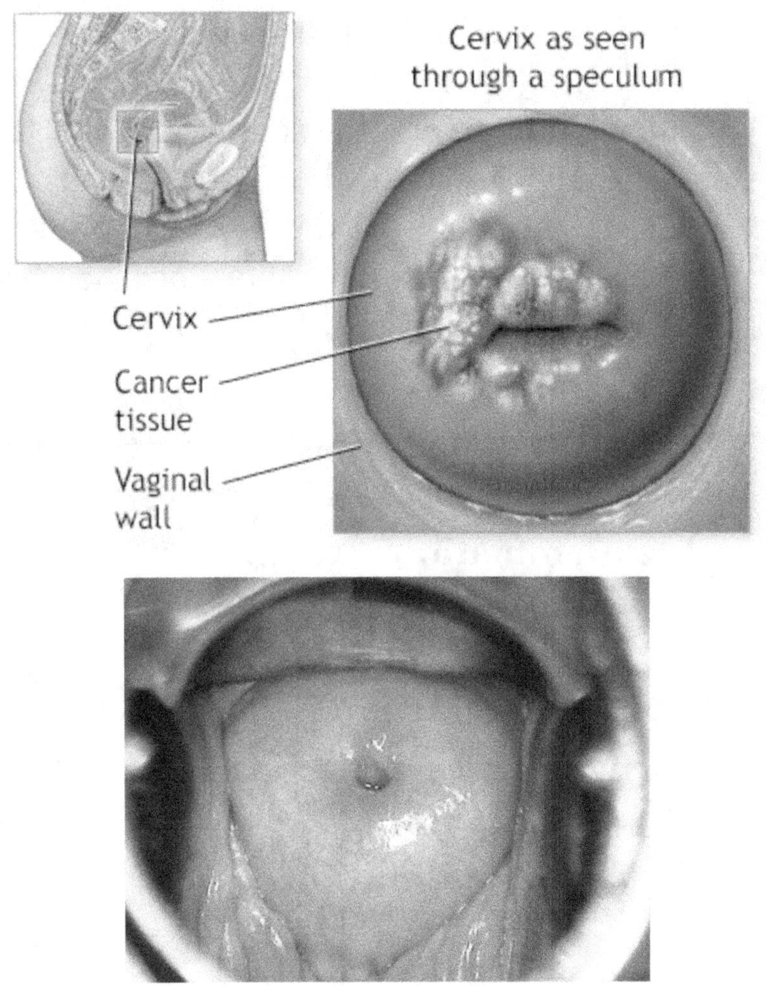

Section 5

Cervical Cancer Diagnosis

Prior to diagnosing cervical cancer, screening tests like a pap smear are conducted to detect early cases of the disease before any symptoms manifest. During this test, a doctor gathers cells from the cervical canal and examines them under a microscope to identify any alterations in the appearance of cervical cells that may indicate the potential development of cervical cancer or signs of HPV infection.The various changes that can be observed include:

- **Normal cells:** Healthy cervical cells with no signs of abnormalities.

- **Inflammation**: Changes in the cells caused by an infection or irritation.

- Atypical squamous cells: Mild changes in the shape and size of squamous cells.

- **High-grade squamous intraepithelial lesion (HSIL):** More severe changes in squamous cells that may indicate pre-cancerous conditions.

- **Low-grade squamous intraepithelial lesion (LSIL):** Minor abnormalities in squamous cells, often associated with HPV infection.

- **Squamous cell cancer:** The presence of cancerous cells in the cervix.

- Adenocarcinoma in situ: Early-stage cancer in the glandular cells of the cervix.

The results of the pap smear guide further diagnostic and treatment decisions. Regular pap smears are essential for early detection and prevention of cervical cancer.

Colposcopy:

A colposcopy is typically performed in conjunction with a PAP smear to visually examine the lower part of the womb for any visible abnormal growth or changes in the cervix.HPV testing: This test is conducted to identify the presence of the human papillomavirus (HPV) and determine the specific strain responsible for the infection. If the infection is caused by HPV strains 6 and 11, the risk of cancer development is low, and it may result in the formation of genital warts, which often resolve on their own. However, if the strain detected is 16 or 18, the risk of malignancy increases, and the patient requires close monitoring.In cases of extensive cervical involvement, the following imaging scans are employed to assess the spread of cancer cells:

- CT scan

- MRI scan

- PET-CT scan

- Chest X-ray

These diagnostic procedures help determine the stage and extent of cervical cancer, guiding appropriate treatment decisions.

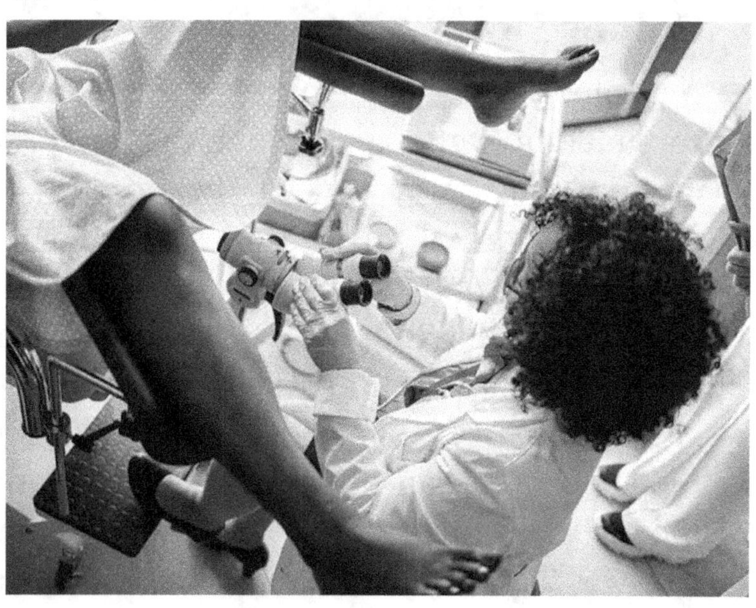

Section 6

Cervical Cancer Treatment - Briefing

The protocol of treatment varies with respect to the stage of cancer development, its spread, size of the portion of cervix involved and the general health of the patient.

- In precancerous stages: Only the affected portion of the cervix is removed usually by laser or diathermy and the rest of the cervix is left as it is.

The commonly used procedures are LLETZ (Laser Loop Excision of the transformation zone) where a heated wire loop is used to remove all the abnormal cells.

The second method used is cone biopsy, where a cone-shaped tissue having abnormal cells is removed.

- In case of invasive cancer, partial removal of the cervix or complete removal of the cervix along with the uterus can be done (hysterectomy).

- In case of systemic metastasis, chemotherapy and radiotherapy are given to kill the distant metastasis cells.

- Lymph nodes may be removed along with the infiltrated organs

- Targeted therapy: Medicines like Avastin (Bevacizumab), which are specially targeted against cervical cancer cells can be given

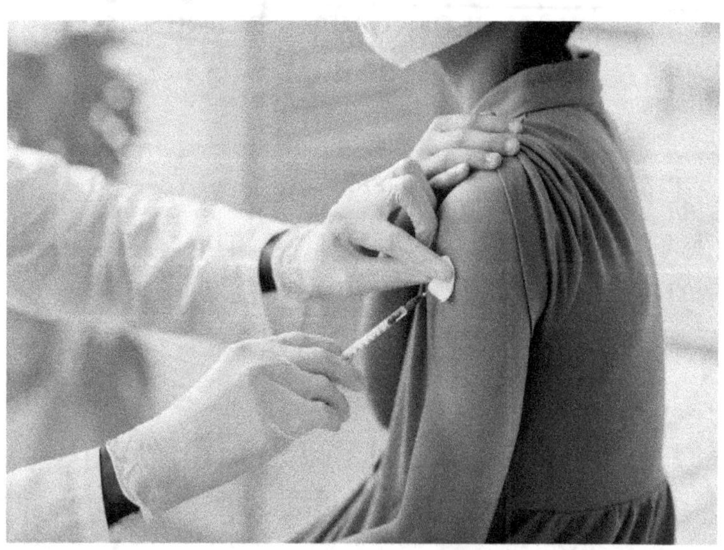

Vaccination Dosage being Administered

Detailed Clinical Approaches to Cervical Cancer Treatment & Management

Immunization

The 9-valent HPV vaccine (Gardasil 9 [9vHPV]) is available in the United States to decrease the risk of certain cancers and precancerous lesions in males and females. The 9vHPV vaccine covers HPV subtypes 6, 11, 16, 18, 31, 33, 45, 52, and 58. Cervarix (2vHPV) and Gardasil (4vHPV) were discontinued in the United States in October 2016.

It is estimated that the 9vHPV vaccine can increase prevention of cervical high-grade squamous intraepithelial lesions in up to 90% of cases compared with the quadrivalent HPV vaccine. [5]

Stage-based treatment

The treatment of cervical cancer varies with the stage of the disease. For early invasive cancer, surgery is the treatment of choice. In more advanced cases, radiation combined with chemotherapy is the current standard of care. In patients with disseminated disease, chemotherapy or radiation provides symptom palliation. The treatment of cervical cancer frequently requires a multidisciplinary approach. Involvement of a gynecologic oncologist, radiation oncologist, and medical oncologist may be necessary.

The treatment of cervical cancer varies with the stage of the disease. For early invasive cancer, surgery is the treatment of choice.

In more advanced cases, radiation combined with chemotherapy is the current standard of care. In patients with disseminated disease, chemotherapy or radiation provides symptom palliation. (See Treatment and Medication.)

Stage-Based Therapy

Stage 0 cancer

Carcinoma in situ (stage 0) is treated with local ablative or excisional measures such as cryosurgery, laser ablation, and loop excision.

Surgical removal is preferred in that it allows further pathologic evaluation to rule out microinvasive disease. After treatment, these patients require lifelong surveillance.

Stage IA1 cancer

The treatment of choice for stage IA1 disease is surgery. Total hysterectomy, radical hysterectomy, and conization are accepted procedures. Lymph node dissection is not required if the depth of invasion is less than 3 mm and no lymphovascular invasion is noted.

Selected patients with stage IA1 disease but no lymphovascular space invasion who desire to maintain fertility may undergo therapeutic conization with close follow-up, including cytology, colposcopy, and endocervical curettage. Patients with comorbid medical conditions who are not surgical candidates can be successfully treated with radiation.

According to National Comprehensive Cancer Network (NCCN) guidelines, pelvic radiation therapy is currently a category 1 recommendation for women with stage IA disease and negative lymph nodes after surgery who have high-risk factors (eg, a large primary tumor, deep stromal invasion, or lymphovascular space invasion).

Stage IA2, IB, or IIA cancer

For patients with stage IB or IIA disease, there are 2 treatment options:

- Combined external beam radiation with brachytherapy
- Radical hysterectomy with bilateral pelvic lymphadenectomy

Radical vaginal trachelectomy with pelvic lymph node dissection is appropriate for fertility preservation in women with stage IA2 disease and those with stage IB1 disease whose lesions are 2 cm or smaller. [6] The principal problems with pregnancy after trachelectomy are premature labor and the need to undergo cesarean section for delivery.

In a retrospective review of 62 patients with stage IB1 cervical carcinoma who underwent attempted radical trachelectomy and underwent preoperative magnetic resonance imaging (MRI), Lakhman et al found that pre trachelectomy MRI helped identify high-risk patients who were likely to need radical hysterectomy and helped confirm the absence of residual tumor after a cone biopsy with negative margins. A tumor size of 2 cm or larger and deep cervical stromal invasion on MRI were associated with an increased chance of radical hysterectomy.

Most retrospective studies have shown equivalent survival rates for trachelectomy and hysterectomy, though such studies usually are flawed because of patient selection bias and other compounding factors. However, a 2008 study showed identical overall and disease-free survival rates for the 2 procedures.

Current surgical guidelines for stage IA2 to IIA cervical cancers allow for minimally invasive techniques, such as traditional laparoscopic and robotically assisted laparoscopic techniques, in the surgical management of these tumors. Indeed, it has been shown that these less morbid procedures are equally effective in achieving adequate surgical margins and lymph node dissection while possessing the added advantage of shorter postoperative recovery times.

An analysis of women from the Surveillance, Epidemiology, and End Results (SEER) database who underwent radical hysterectomy with lymphadenectomy revealed that patients with node-negative early-stage cervical cancer who underwent a more extensive lymphadenectomy had improved survival. Compared with patients who had fewer than 10 nodes removed, patients who had 21-30 nodes removed were 24% less likely to die of their tumors, and those who had more than 30 nodes removed were 37% less likely to die.

Postoperative irradiation of the pelvis reduces the risk of local recurrence in patients with high-risk factors (ie, positive pelvic nodes, positive surgical margins, and residual parametrial disease). A randomized trial showed that patients with parametrial involvement, positive pelvic nodes, or positive surgical margins benefit from a postoperative combination of cisplatin-containing chemotherapy and pelvic irradiation. Postoperative radiation therapy is also recommended in patients who have at least 2 intermediate risk factors (including tumor size greater than 2 cm, deep stromal invasion, or lymphovascular space invasion). For patients with IB2 or IIA cancer and tumors larger than 4 cm, radiation and chemotherapy is selected in most cases. Risks are associated with combined therapy, but many of these patients will meet either intermediate- or high-risk criteria after radical hysterectomy and therefore are strong candidates for this approach.

Stage IIB, III, or IVA cancer

For locally advanced cervical carcinoma (stages IIB, III, and IVA), radiation therapy was the treatment of choice for many years. Radiation therapy begins with a course of external beam radiation to reduce tumor mass and thereby enable subsequent intracavitary application. Brachytherapy is delivered by means of afterloading applicators that are placed in the uterine cavity and vagina.

Additionally, the results from large, well-conducted, prospective randomized clinical trials have demonstrated a dramatic improvement in survival when chemotherapy is combined with radiation therapy. Consequently, the use of cisplatin-based chemotherapy in combination with radiation has become the standard of care for primary management of patients with locally advanced cervical cancer.

Stage IVB and recurrent cancer

Individualized therapy is used on a palliative basis. Radiation therapy is used alone for control of bleeding and pain, whereas systemic chemotherapy is used for disseminated disease. For recurrent disease, the choice of therapy is influenced by the treatments previously employed.

Treatment of pelvic recurrences after primary surgical management should include single-agent chemotherapy and radiation, and treatment for recurrences elsewhere should include combination chemotherapy. For central pelvic recurrence after radiation therapy, modified radical hysterectomy (if the recurrence is smaller than 2 cm) or pelvic exenteration should be undertaken.

For disease recurring after chemotherapy and radiation therapy, a disease-free interval of more than 16 months is considered to designate the tumor as platinum-sensitive. The standard of care in these cases is chemotherapy with a platinum-based doublet of paclitaxel and cisplatin.

The NCCN also recommends docetaxel, gemcitabine, ifosfamide, 5-fluorouracil, mitomycin, irinotecan, and topotecan as possible candidates for second-line therapy (category 2B recommendation), as well as pemetrexed and vinorelbine (category 3 recommendation). In addition, bevacizumab as single-agent therapy is also acceptable.

Treatment with bevacizumab plus cisplatin and paclitaxel or topotecan and paclitaxel was approved by the FDA in August 2014 for persistent, recurrent, or metastatic cervical cancer. A statistically significant improvement in overall survival (OS) and an increase in the rate of tumor shrinkage was shown in women treated with bevacizumab plus chemotherapy compared with chemotherapy alone.

However, hypertension, thromboembolic events, and GI fistulas were higher in the bevacizumab group. Bevacizumab/paclitaxel/cisplatin or topotecan is considered a first-line regimen for recurrent or metastatic cervical cancer.

Recurrences arising in a previously irradiated field or after a disease-free interval of less than 16 months are less likely to respond to subsequent therapies. Consequently, patients with such recurrences should be strongly encouraged to participate in clinical trials. Special efforts should be made to ensure that they receive comprehensive palliative care, including adequate pain control.

In June 2018, the FDA approved pembrolizumab for treatment of recurrent or metastatic cervical cancer with disease progression on or after chemotherapy in patients whose tumors express PD-L1 (CPS 1 or greater) as determined by an FDA-approved test. Approval was based on the KEYNOTE-158 clinical trial (n=98). For the 77 patients whose tumors expressed PD-L1 with a complete response rate (CRR) of 1 or greater, the overall response rate (ORR) was 14.3%, with a CRR of 2.6% and partial response rate of 11.7%. Among the 11 responding patients, median duration of response (DoR) was not yet reached (range, 4.1 to 18.6+ months), and 91% experienced a DoR of 6 months or longer. The median follow-up time was 11.7 months (range, 0.6 to 22.7 months).

Pembrolizumab was also granted accelerated approval for unresectable or metastatic tumor mutational burden-high (TMB-H) [≥10 mutations/megabase (mut/Mb)] solid tumors in patients that have progressed following prior treatment and who have no alternative treatment options.

Approval was based on results in a prospectively-planned retrospective analysis of 10 cohorts of previously treated patients with various unresectable or metastatic TMB-H solid tumors enrolled in a multicenter, nonrandomized, open-label trial, KEYNOTE-158. Among the 13% of patients identified as TMB-H, defined as TMB ≥10 mut/Mb, the ORR for these patients was 29%, with a 4% CRR and 25% partial response rate. The median DoR was not reached, with 57% of patients having response durations ≥12 months and 50% of patients having response durations ≥24 months. [93]

Complications of Therapy

- **Radiation-related complications:** During the acute phase of pelvic radiation therapy, the surrounding normal tissues (eg, intestines, bladder, and perineal skin) often are affected. Acute adverse gastrointestinal (GI) effects include diarrhea, abdominal cramping, rectal discomfort, and bleeding. Diarrhea can usually be controlled by giving either loperamide or atropine sulfate. Small steroid-containing enemas are prescribed to alleviate symptoms from proctitis. Cystourethritis also can occur, leading to dysuria, frequency, and nocturia. Antispasmodics often are helpful for symptom relief. Urine should be examined for possible infection. If urinary tract infection (UTI) is diagnosed, therapy should be instituted without delay. Proper skin hygiene should be maintained for the perineum. Topical lotion should be used if erythema or desquamation occurs. Late sequelae of radiation therapy usually appear 1-4 years after treatment. The major sequelae include rectal or vaginal stenosis, small bowel obstruction, malabsorption, radiation enteritis, and chronic cystitis.

- **Surgical complications:** The most frequent complication of radical hysterectomy is urinary dysfunction resulting from partial denervation of the detrusor muscle. Other complications include foreshortened vagina, ureterovaginal fistula, hemorrhage, infection, bowel obstruction, stricture and fibrosis of the intestine or rectosigmoid colon, and bladder and rectovaginal fistulas. Invasive procedures (eg, nephrostomy or diverting colostomy) sometimes are performed in this group of patients to improve their quality of life.

Nutrition

Proper nutrition is important for patients with cervical cancer. Every attempt should be made to encourage and provide adequate oral food intake. Nutritional supplements (eg, Ensure [Abbott Nutrition, Columbus, OH] or Boost [Nestlé HealthCare Nutrition, Fremont, MI]) are used when patients have had significant weight loss or cannot tolerate regular food because of nausea caused by radiation or chemotherapy. In patients with severe anorexia, appetite stimulants such as megestrol can be prescribed.

For patients who are unable to tolerate any oral intake, percutaneous endoscopic gastrostomy tubes are placed for nutritional supplementation. In patients with extensive bowel obstruction as a result of metastatic cancer, hyperalimentation sometimes is used.

Prevention of Human Papillomavirus Infection

Human papillomavirus (HPV) infection is usually transmitted sexually, though rare cases have been reported in virgins. Condom use may not prevent transmission. A study in a mouse model by Roberts et al found that a widely used vaginal spermicide, nonoxynol-9, greatly increased susceptibility to HPV infection, whereas carrageenan, a polysaccharide present in some vaginal lubricants, prevented infection.

One HPV vaccine is available in the United States. A nine-valent HPV vaccine (Gardasil 9, 9vHPV) is indicated for females aged 9 through 45 years to prevent cervical cancer (and also genital warts and anal cancer); in addition to coverage of HPV types 6, 11, 16, and 18, it covers HPV types 31, 33, 45, 52, and 58. Other HPV vaccines (2vHPV [Cervarix], 4vHPV [Gardasil]) are no longer available in the United States.

The 9vHPV vaccine is approved by the FDA for routine HPV vaccination of females and males aged 9 through 45 years.The vaccination series can be started as young as age 9 years. Catch-up vaccination is recommended for females aged 13-26 years who have not been previously vaccinated or who have not completed the full series. The 9vHPV vaccine may be offered as a 2-dose series for children and young adolescents aged 9-14 years.

Screening for cervical cancer should continue in vaccinated women, following the same guidelines as in unvaccinated women. [3] These vaccines do not provide complete protection against cervical cancer; oncogenic HPV types other than 16 and 18 account for about 30% of cases, and cross-protection may be only partial. In addition, not all vaccinated patients may mount an effective response to the vaccine, particularly if they do not receive all 3 doses or if they get the doses at time intervals that are not associated with efficacy.

Finally, the duration of protection with these vaccines has not yet been determined. The available evidence suggests that immunity from infection with the HPV types covered by these vaccines will persist for at least 6-8 years, but continuing follow-up will be required to determine whether revaccination will be necessary.

The safety of HPV vaccines is a deeply controversial topic. Follow-up of large patient populations who participated in phase 3 clinical trials has documented that both FDA-approved HPV vaccines are extremely safe. Articles in the popular media, however, have detailed cases of young women with devastating illnesses attributed to the vaccines.

In post licensure safety surveillance for the quadrivalent HPV vaccine, 6.2% of all reports to the Vaccine Adverse Event Reporting System (VAERS) described serious adverse events, including neurologic injury (eg, Guillain-Barré syndrome) and 32 reports of death. In comparison with other vaccines, rates of most of these adverse events were no greater than the background rates, but there was disproportionate reporting of syncope and venous thromboembolic events.

Section 7

Prevention of Cervical Cancer

A person contracts cervical cancer due to a long-term infection by the human papillomavirus (HPV), a virus that is usually transmitted from one person to another via sexual activity or even skin-to-skin contact. HPV is a common type of sexually transmitted infection (STI) with over 30 different strains that can affect a human's genitals. While many persons who are sexually active are at risk of having HPV, only a very small number of them will eventually be diagnosed with cervical cancer.

The best way to treat cervical cancer promptly is to detect it early via cervical screenings. Early vaccination with the HPV vaccine also improves a person's odds in the long term.

Beyond early screenings and vaccination, what else can you do to take care of your cervix? Sometimes, even simple steps and lifestyle modifications can go a long way to safeguarding your cervix's health.

Below are Some factors thought to lower the chances of cancer development like:

- HPV vaccine (Bivalent, Quadrivalent, and multivalent vaccines against various subtypes of HPV are known to significantly reduce the risk of cancer development)

- Healthy diet maintenance

- Practice safe sex with the use of condoms

- Practice safe sex: Using a condom during sexual activity helps to lower the risk of getting or spreading HPV.

- Limit the number of sexual partners: You can still be at higher risk of contracting HPV.

- Quit smoking: Smoking is a known risk factor that can cause cervical cancer; smokers are twice as likely to get cervical cancer compared to non-smokers.

- Get tested for STIs: STIs also may not cause symptoms, so regular screenings can be helpful to prevent any future risk of cervical cancer. If you are worried that you or your partner may have an STI, or if you did not practice safe sex, consider getting screened immediately.

- Follow-up appointments: Be sure not to miss these, as follow-up procedures can be beneficial in catching warning signs early before it gets serious. Make sure to follow the doctor's advice and ask questions if you need clarification on anything.

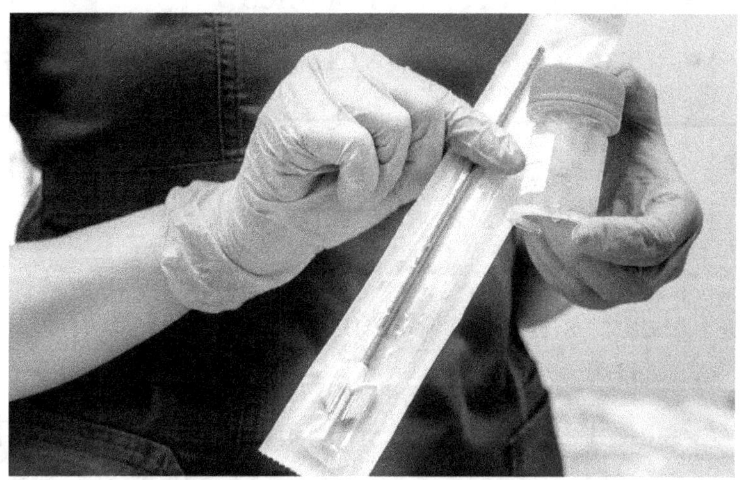

Cervical Cancer screening: the Current state of testing.

Section 8

Myths and Facts about Cervical Cancer

Despite a growing awareness of the nature of cervical cancer, some segments of society continue to carry on the myths and misconceptions about cervical cancer, especially with regard to persons diagnosed with it.

Stigma Towards Survivors

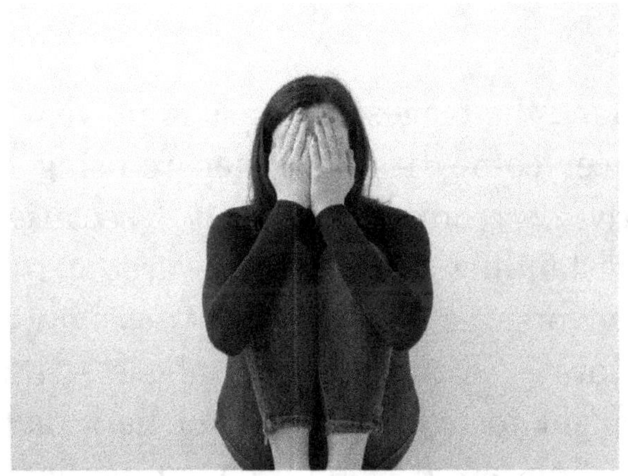

Much of the stigma towards cervical cancer survivors stems from the association of the HPV virus with sexual activity.

For most people, the assumption is that having HPV is a sure sign of promiscuity and/or infidelity. As a result, women are at risk of being shunned or abused by others should the nature of their illness be known.

Many women may refuse to go for cervical screening, even if they are not actually at risk of developing the condition, all because the association of a screening automatically puts them in a "shameful" position.

Much of the stigma directed toward survivors stems from a lack of awareness and understanding of cervical cancer.

In fact, the biggest obstacle to preventing cervical cancer comes from women refusing to undergo early screenings, mainly because of the longstanding prejudices towards cervical cancer survivors, as well as the possibility of other factors – such as sexual abuse – that are not brought to light. It does not help that a routine question asked when a person is diagnosed with cervical cancer is "How many sexual partners have you had?"

It is therefore critical to improving society's awareness of cervical cancer in order to do away with the stigmatization that has occurred for so long. Programs such as medical literacy campaigns are but a few ways to tackle the root of the problem head-on.

Myth 1:

Having HPV Guarantees a Cervical Cancer Diagnosis

Fact: Not true

- *There are many different types of HPV, but not all of them cause cervical cancer. In some cases, your immune system can get rid of the virus within one to two years or so. 80 to 90 per cent of women will not suffer any long-term complications. Other than that, the HPV virus may persist and become dormant, lingering in a person's body for some time before it starts causing cells in the cervix to multiply uncontrollably. For the most part, changes caused by HPV happen without you realizing it until you get screened. If left untreated, these changes can eventually cause cervical cancer.*

Myth 2:

Cervical Cancer is Inherited

Fact: Not true

- *Unlike breast or ovarian cancer, cervical cancer is not hereditary. It is caused primarily by the HPV virus. Early screenings and HPV vaccinations for children are the best ways to prevent the disease from occurring/advancing.*

Myth 3:

Only Women with Multiple Partners Get Cervical Cancer

Fact: Not true

- *This particularly long-lived myth has been a strong source of stigmatization towards survivors. The main cause of cervical cancer is HPV, which can still spread to a person even if they only have one partner or are not very sexually active. As long as the HPV persists in the body for a long time, it can eventually progress the abnormalities in the cervix into cervical cancer. Safe sex does protect you from the risk of contracting HPV, but any unprotected skin can still allow HPV to transmit itself to another person (since the virus spreads from skin-to-skin contact).*

Myth 4:

No Screenings Needed for Those Who are Vaccinated/Not Sexually Active

Fact: Not true

- *Those with HPV may not show any symptoms (asymptomatic cases), making it difficult to tell if a person is at risk of cervical cancer or not. Through cervical screening, doctors can look for signs or markers of any abnormalities in your cervix, and take the necessary action to prevent it from spreading or mitigating whatever damage it has caused to the body. Despite the HPV vaccine proving effective at protecting young girls from HPV, regular screenings are still recommended, especially as the vaccine does not protect you from all forms of HPV. It's also important to remember that not all HPVs cause cancer. Regardless, a woman can still be at risk of contracting a cancer-causing type of HPV before receiving the vaccine.*

Myth 5:
Cervical Cancer Cannot Be Prevented
Fact: Not true

- *Early cervical screenings and HPV vaccinations are the most effective ways of prevention, either detecting an HPV infection before it can progress into cervical cancer or preventing it at an early age. HPV may cause some complications that can be addressed with medication but can be prevented through the HPV vaccine.*

Myth 6:

Cervical Screenings are Painful

Fact: Not true

- *A cervical screening's purpose is to find any precancerous cell changes in the cervix. It involves a test to look for any HPV infections or a Pap test (also called a Pap smear) that takes a sample of cervical cells to look for signs that could lead to cervical cancer; in some cases, a co-test involving both tests may be done. The screening involves the use of a device called a speculum, which a doctor will use to gently open your vagina to inspect the cervix. A soft, narrow brush or a spatula-like instrument may be used to collect cellular samples, which are sent to the lab for testing. When the speculum is used, some women may experience some discomfort. If you feel any pain, be sure to let the accompanying nurse (or the doctor) know and they will do what they can to help ease the pain; if need be, they will use a smaller speculum. The procedure only takes up to 30 seconds to complete, and you'll be notified every step of the way about what they are doing to help alleviate any concerns you might have. You can also request to stop the procedure if you feel uncomfortable or are experiencing any pain. As part of its mission, the ROSE Foundation has introduced a do-it-yourself screening test that only takes five minutes to complete. This self-test is a simple, convenient procedure you can do on your own with minimal fuss and no pain, and you'll be able to get the results within three weeks.*

Myth 7:

Cervical Screenings Also Detect Other Cancers

Fact: Not true

- *1 in 5 people mistakenly believe that a cervical screening detects ovarian cancer or other types of STIs. The reality is that cervical screenings are preventive tools to detect abnormal cellular changes in the cervix at an early stage that could cause cervical cancer.*

Myth 8:

Cervical Screenings Protect Women from Cervical Cancer

Fact: Partly true

- *Cervical screenings are an effective method to reduce a person's risk of cervical cancer. It's important to note that you can take steps to greatly reduce the risk of cervical cancer, but preventing HPV infections is not as easy. Vaccines do protect you from HPV, but not from all types of high-risk HPVs. You can consider cervical screenings and HPV vaccination as the first line of defense against cervical cancer.*

Myth 9:

Cervical Cancer Survivors Cannot Get Pregnant

Fact: Not true

- *HPV infections can potentially complicate a pregnancy, but it does not affect a person's ability to conceive. If, however, there is a need to remove abnormal cells in the cervix, that could affect your ability to conceive or reach a full term in your pregnancy. Again, this does not cause infertility.*

Myth 10:

Cervical Cancer Causes Symptoms

Fact: Not true

- *In a majority of cases, people with an HPV infection do not show any signs or symptoms, and the infection will go away on its own after some time. Even if it develops into cervical cancer, you may not have any symptoms at all until the disease advances. It is why early screenings are very important to prevent cervical cancer: the earlier you get screened, the earlier doctors can detect signs of cervical cancer and take the necessary course of action to treat it before it worsens.*

Myth 11:

Cervical Screenings are Needed Every Year

Fact: Partly true

- The frequency of screenings depends on a few factors, such as your age, your health condition, and whether you've previously had an HPV infection. However, you don't necessarily need to go for a screening every year. If you are at higher risk of contracting HPV, you may need more frequent screenings as set by your doctor. But even if you don't fall into the high-risk category, regular screenings are still recommended.

Myth 12:

Cervical Cancer Only Happens in Less Developed Countries

Fact: Not true

- HPV infections and cervical cancer can affect anyone, regardless of age, gender, affluence, social standing, or education level.

First Steps to Taking Care of Your Cervical Health

It becomes essential for women to take good care of their cervical health. Again, we cannot understate how important both the HPV vaccination and early cervical screenings can be in protecting you and your loved ones from cervical cancer. Even if the vaccination does not provide comprehensive coverage against all types of HPV, it nevertheless protects you and your loved ones from the most common types of HPV which causes cervical cancer. Any level of protection is still necessary for long-term prevention.

Awareness is also very important to ensure that fewer women get cervical cancer later in life. With January being Cervical Health Awareness Month, this is the perfect time to raise awareness about HPV and cervical cancer. Each and every person plays a role in debunking myths that only serve to prevent women from getting life-saving early screenings and vaccinations. As long as these myths continue to perpetuate stigmas toward cervical cancer survivors, it will be difficult to achieve the elimination of cervical cancer in the country. Better health literacy can go a long way toward helping women take better care of their cervical health while also contributing to the elimination of cervical cancer in time.

Section 9

FAQs on Cervical Cancer

Do the symptoms of cervical cancer manifest suddenly?

The symptoms of cervical cancer typically do not appear suddenly. However, once these symptoms begin, they tend to persist. In many cases, cervical cancer is asymptomatic, but some women may eventually experience abnormal vaginal bleeding, unusual vaginal discharge, pain during sexual intercourse, pelvic or lower back pain, swelling in the legs, and more.

Cervical cancer is a significant concern among gynecologic cancers on a global scale. According to research published in 2022, it ranks fourteenth among all cancer types and is the fourth most prevalent cancer among women worldwide. In this article, we'll explore whether the symptoms of cervical cancer suddenly appear and if it can be detected in its early stages.

Can cervical cancer be detected in its early stages?

Early stages of cervical cancer are typically asymptomatic, making it challenging to diagnose. The first signs of cervical cancer often take several years to develop. Cervical cancer tends to grow slowly, and its malignancy can increase over time. The progression from precancerous cells to cervical cancer is a gradual process, and it can take years for human papillomavirus (HPV) infection to lead to cervical cancer.

The most effective way to detect cervical cancer in its early stages is through regular screening tests. Screening tests, such as the HPV test and Pap test, can identify abnormal cells and aid in early diagnosis. In some cases, both the HPV and Pap tests are performed together, referred to as a co-test. Early detection is crucial for timely medical intervention.

Can cervical cancer develop within a year?

Cervical cancer is typically not a condition that develops within a year. It's a cancer that can affect many women at some point in their lives. Cervical cancer is primarily caused by the human papillomavirus (HPV), which is a sexually transmitted infection. It's important to note that cervical cancer is not hereditary and is not passed from parents to children. Maintaining a healthy sexual routine can help reduce the risk of cervical cancer.

How quickly does cervical cancer progress?

Cervical cancer progresses slowly, and its malignancy tends to increase over time. The development of toxic cells into cervical cancer is a gradual process. It takes several years for human papillomavirus (HPV) to lead to cervical cancer.

Changes in the cervix can begin as early as a woman's 20s or 30s, but the actual diagnosis may not occur until her 50s. This slow progression allows for opportunities for early detection and treatment. Therefore, it's crucial for women to have regular health checkups to identify any abnormal changes as soon as possible. The Pap (Papanicolaou) Test is a helpful tool for doctors in suspecting cervical cancer. Additionally, women should be aware of any unusual symptoms that would warrant a prompt visit to a doctor.

Can cervical cancer cause infertility?

Yes, cervical cancer can lead to infertility. The cancer itself can spread to the uterus, impacting fertility. Additionally, the treatments for cervical cancer, such as surgery and radiotherapy, can also result in infertility. For instance, a radical hysterectomy, which is a surgical procedure to remove the womb, can make it challenging to conceive. Furthermore, radiotherapy can harm the uterus and interfere with egg production in the ovaries. These factors combined can make it difficult or even impossible for women with cervical cancer to have children.

Can I have a baby if I have cervical cancer?

In some cases, yes. Surgeries such as cone biopsy and radical trachelectomy can enable women with cervical cancer to have a baby. Cone biopsy involves the removal of the affected cervical tissues, while radical trachelectomy entails removing most of the cervix and the upper part of the vagina. Additionally, a stitch is placed around the internal opening of the cervix to close it permanently. These procedures can facilitate pregnancy, but there is a slightly elevated risk of premature birth or having a baby with low birth weight.

Can the symptoms of cervical cancer make pregnancy difficult?

It's possible. The symptoms of cervical cancer can make it challenging to maintain a pregnancy. Cervical cancer can cause abnormal vaginal bleeding, an unusual discharge from the vagina, pain during sex, pelvic pain, leg swelling, irregular urination or bowel movements, and blood in the urine. These symptoms and the condition itself may impact a pregnancy.

Are cervical cancer tumors visible or felt during general checkups, or can a doctor detect them in routine physical examinations?

It's possible, but typically, cervical cancer tumors are only felt or seen at advanced stages. During early stages, they often go unnoticed as they don't present visible or palpable symptoms.

Cervical cancer often remains undiagnosed, particularly in its early stages. The most common risk factor for cervical cancer is the human papillomavirus (HPV), which is sexually transmitted and can lead to cervical intraepithelial neoplasia and invasive cervical cancer. This article explores whether cervical cancer tumors can be detected during general checkups.

Can cancer be detected in routine general checkups?

Yes, it is possible. A routine pelvic examination can raise suspicion of cancer. During a pelvic exam, the doctor assesses the reproductive organs. People often undergo regular pelvic checkups or exams based on their doctor's recommendations, particularly if they have symptoms such as unusual vaginal discharge or pelvic pain. If cervical cancer is suspected, the doctor may request a Pap test following the pelvic exam.

A Pap test is a valuable tool for initiating the examination of cancer. It can help reduce the number of undiagnosed cases by identifying potential issues early.

Again, in the advanced stages of cervical cancer, a tumor or growth may be visible during general physical checkups. However, this is not the case in the early stages. Cervical cancer often goes unnoticed during the early stages because it typically doesn't present symptoms. During a pelvic and vaginal examination, a doctor can detect any abnormal growth by examining the vulva, vagina, cervix, ovaries, uterus, rectum, and pelvis within a few minutes. However, it's important to note that a pelvic exam and a Pap test together only help a doctor suspect cervical cancer and are not definitive diagnostic tests for every individual.

www.ingramcontent.com/pod-product-compliance
Lightning Source LLC
Chambersburg PA
CBHW070727260726
48660CB00007B/2759